HOW TO IMPROVE YOUR HEALTH

How to Improve Your Health
Walter the Educator

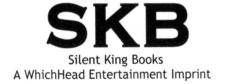

Silent King Books
A WhichHead Entertainment Imprint

How to Improve Your Health is a little problem solver book by Walter the Educator that belongs to the Little Problem Solver Books Series.
Collect them all and more books at WaltertheEducator.com

LITTLE PROBLEM
SOLVER BOOKS

INTRO

In the modern world, where stress, processed foods, and sedentary lifestyles are common, maintaining good health is more critical than ever. Your health is the foundation of your life, and improving it requires deliberate actions across multiple dimensions, including physical fitness, nutrition, mental well-being, and lifestyle choices. While health can be complex, achieving and maintaining it can be simplified by understanding key principles and implementing practical strategies. In this little book, we will explore comprehensive ways to improve your health, ranging from physical activity, diet, and mental wellness, to sleep, hydration, and personal habits.

How to Improve Your Health

The Importance of Physical Fitness

Regular physical activity is one of the most effective ways to improve your overall health. Exercise not only enhances your physical condition but also has significant mental and emotional benefits. Many people think that being physically fit means having a gym membership or running marathons, but physical fitness encompasses a wide variety of activities and is achievable for people of all fitness levels.

How to Improve Your Health

1. Cardiovascular Exercise Cardiovascular or aerobic exercise is essential for improving the health of your heart and lungs. Activities such as walking, running, swimming, cycling, and dancing increase your heart rate and improve circulation. Cardiovascular exercises are also effective for burning calories, reducing body fat, and increasing endurance.

How to Improve Your Health

The Centers for Disease Control and Prevention (CDC) recommend that adults engage in at least 150 minutes of moderate-intensity aerobic activity per week. This can be broken down into manageable increments, such as 30 minutes a day, five days a week.

How to Improve Your Health

2. Strength Training In addition to cardiovascular exercise, strength training is vital for building muscle mass, improving bone density, and boosting metabolism. Strength training can be done using weights, resistance bands, or even your own body weight through exercises like push-ups, squats, and lunges.

How to Improve Your Health

It's important to include strength training in your fitness routine at least two to three times per week. Stronger muscles not only improve physical appearance but also enhance functional fitness, which means performing everyday tasks with ease.

How to Improve Your Health

3. Flexibility and Balance Flexibility and balance are often overlooked but are critical components of overall physical health, especially as we age. Stretching exercises such as yoga or Pilates improve flexibility, which can prevent injury and reduce muscle stiffness.

How to Improve Your Health

Balance exercises help in maintaining coordination and preventing falls, particularly in older adults. Incorporating stretching and balance exercises into your routine can enhance mobility, posture, and body alignment.

How to Improve Your Health

4. Consistency and Enjoyment While exercise is important, consistency is key to seeing long-term benefits. To improve your health, it's important to find physical activities that you enjoy. Whether it's hiking, dancing, swimming, or cycling, when you enjoy your exercise routine, you're more likely to stick with it. Make fitness a regular part of your life rather than a temporary goal.

How to Improve Your Health

Nutrition: Fueling Your Body for Optimal Health

Nutrition plays a pivotal role in improving and maintaining your health. The food you eat provides the essential nutrients your body needs to function optimally. However, with so much conflicting information about diets and eating plans, it can be overwhelming to know where to start.

How to Improve Your Health

1. The Importance of a Balanced Diet A balanced diet includes a variety of foods from all the major food groups: fruits, vegetables, lean proteins, whole grains, and healthy fats. Each of these food groups provides specific nutrients that your body requires.

How to Improve Your Health

For example, fruits and vegetables are rich in vitamins, minerals, and antioxidants that help protect your cells and support immune function. Lean proteins, such as chicken, fish, beans, and tofu, are necessary for muscle repair and growth. Whole grains provide fiber, which aids digestion and keeps blood sugar levels stable.

How to Improve Your Health

2. Macronutrients: Carbohydrates, Proteins, and Fats

Understanding macronutrients—carbohydrates, proteins, and fats—is key to improving your health through nutrition.

How to Improve Your Health

- **Carbohydrates:** Carbohydrates are your body's primary source of energy. However, it's important to choose complex carbohydrates, such as whole grains, fruits, and vegetables, over simple carbohydrates like sugar and refined grains, which can lead to weight gain and blood sugar spikes.

How to Improve Your Health

- **Proteins:** Protein is essential for muscle growth, tissue repair, and immune function. It is found in meat, poultry, fish, eggs, legumes, and plant-based sources like lentils and quinoa.

How to Improve Your Health

- **Fats:** Healthy fats, such as those found in olive oil, avocados, nuts, and fatty fish, are essential for brain health, hormone production, and the absorption of fat-soluble vitamins (A, D, E, K). Avoid trans fats and limit saturated fats, which can increase the risk of heart disease.

How to Improve Your Health

3. Micronutrients: Vitamins and Minerals Micronutrients, which include vitamins and minerals, are just as important as macronutrients. These nutrients support various bodily functions, from bone health (calcium, vitamin D) to immune function (vitamin C, zinc).

How to Improve Your Health

A diet rich in fruits and vegetables typically provides the necessary vitamins and minerals your body needs. However, in some cases, supplementation may be necessary to fill gaps in your diet, especially for nutrients like vitamin D, which many people lack.

How to Improve Your Health

4. Hydration Water is critical for nearly every bodily function, including digestion, nutrient transport, and temperature regulation. Drinking enough water each day is one of the simplest ways to improve your health.

How to Improve Your Health

The general recommendation is to drink at least eight 8-ounce glasses of water a day, though individual needs may vary depending on activity level, climate, and overall health. Staying hydrated can improve energy levels, mental clarity, and physical performance.

How to Improve Your Health

5. Mindful Eating In addition to what you eat, how you eat also affects your health. Mindful eating encourages you to pay attention to your hunger and fullness cues, eat slowly, and enjoy your meals without distractions. This practice can help prevent overeating, reduce stress, and enhance your relationship with food.

How to Improve Your Health

Mental Health and Emotional Well-being

Mental health is an integral part of overall well-being, yet it is often neglected in conversations about improving health. Your mental state can impact your physical health and vice versa, making it important to prioritize emotional and psychological wellness.

How to Improve Your Health

1. Managing Stress Chronic stress has been linked to a host of health problems, including heart disease, high blood pressure, digestive issues, and weakened immune function. Finding healthy ways to manage stress is crucial for improving your health. Techniques such as meditation, deep breathing exercises, mindfulness, and journaling can help reduce stress and promote relaxation.

How to Improve Your Health

2. Emotional Resilience Emotional resilience is the ability to bounce back from challenges and maintain mental well-being even in the face of adversity.

How to Improve Your Health

Building emotional resilience involves developing a positive mindset, practicing gratitude, and learning coping strategies to deal with difficult emotions. Seeking support from friends, family, or a therapist when needed is also important for maintaining emotional health.

How to Improve Your Health

3. Social Connections Humans are social creatures, and maintaining strong social connections is vital for mental and emotional health. Studies have shown that people with close relationships are generally happier, healthier, and live longer.

How to Improve Your Health

Make time for meaningful relationships, whether with family, friends, or a supportive community. Social support can buffer against stress, improve mood, and even lower the risk of mental health issues such as depression and anxiety.

How to Improve Your Health

4. Mental Health Awareness Part of improving your mental health involves being aware of your emotional state and recognizing when you might need professional help. Mental health disorders, such as depression, anxiety, and bipolar disorder, are common and treatable.

How to Improve Your Health

If you are struggling with persistent feelings of sadness, hopelessness, or overwhelming stress, seeking help from a mental health professional can be a critical step toward improving your overall well-being.

How to Improve Your Health

The Role of Sleep in Health Improvement

Sleep is often overlooked in discussions about health, but it is just as important as diet and exercise. Poor sleep can negatively affect every aspect of your life, from cognitive function and mood to physical performance and immune system health.

How to Improve Your Health

1. The Importance of Sleep Sleep is the time when your body repairs itself, consolidates memories, and processes emotions. Without adequate sleep, you are more likely to experience fatigue, difficulty concentrating, irritability, and weakened immune function.

How to Improve Your Health

Chronic sleep deprivation has been linked to a higher risk of health problems, including obesity, diabetes, heart disease, and mental health disorders.

How to Improve Your Health

2. Creating a Sleep Routine To improve your sleep and, by extension, your health, it's important to establish a regular sleep routine. This means going to bed and waking up at the same time each day, even on weekends. Creating a relaxing bedtime ritual, such as reading, meditating, or taking a warm bath, can signal to your body that it's time to wind down.

How to Improve Your Health

3. Sleep Environment Your sleep environment also plays a crucial role in the quality of your rest. Make sure your bedroom is cool, dark, and quiet. Investing in a comfortable mattress and pillows can also improve your sleep quality. Avoid using electronic devices like phones, tablets, and computers right before bed, as the blue light emitted by these screens can interfere with your ability to fall asleep.

How to Improve Your Health

4. Prioritizing Rest In a world that values productivity and hustle, it can be tempting to sacrifice sleep for work or entertainment. However, making sleep a priority is one of the best things you can do for your health. Aim for seven to nine hours of sleep per night, and listen to your body's signals when it needs rest.

How to Improve Your Health

Lifestyle Changes for Long-Term Health

Improving your health requires not just short-term efforts but long-term lifestyle changes. Making gradual, sustainable changes to your habits is more effective than drastic, temporary measures.

How to Improve Your Health

1. Avoiding Harmful Habits To improve your health, it's important to avoid or reduce harmful habits such as smoking, excessive alcohol consumption, and drug use. These behaviors increase the risk of various diseases, including cancer, liver disease, and heart disease. Quitting smoking, limiting alcohol intake, and avoiding recreational drugs are crucial steps toward improving both your short-term and long-term health.

How to Improve Your Health

2. Moderation and Balance Living a healthy life doesn't mean depriving yourself of the things you enjoy. Instead, focus on moderation and balance. For example, it's okay to indulge in your favorite treats occasionally, as long as they don't become a regular part of your diet. Balance indulgences with healthier choices and stay mindful of portion sizes.

How to Improve Your Health

3. Time Management and Stress Reduction Modern life is often busy and stressful, making it difficult to prioritize health. Learning to manage your time effectively and reduce unnecessary stress can improve your overall well-being. Incorporate relaxation and leisure activities into your daily schedule, and remember that self-care is essential for both physical and mental health.

How to Improve Your Health

OUTRO

Improving your health is a multifaceted journey that requires a balanced approach to physical fitness, nutrition, mental wellness, sleep, and lifestyle choices. By incorporating regular exercise, eating a nutrient-rich diet, managing stress, fostering emotional well-being, getting enough sleep, and making healthy lifestyle choices, you can significantly improve your overall health and quality of life. Each aspect of health is interconnected, and by focusing on these key areas, you can create lasting positive changes that will benefit you in both the short and long term. Remember that health is not a destination but a continuous process of growth and improvement. Make small, sustainable changes today, and over time, you will see significant improvements in your physical, mental, and emotional well-being.

ABOUT THE CREATOR

Walter the Educator is one of the pseudonyms for Walter Anderson. Formally educated in Chemistry, Business, and Education, he is an educator, an author, a diverse entrepreneur, and he is the son of a disabled war veteran. "Walter the Educator" shares his time between educating and creating. He holds interests and owns several creative projects that entertain, enlighten, enhance, and educate, hoping to inspire and motivate you. Follow, find new works, and stay up to date with Walter the Educator™

at WaltertheEducator.com